Workers' Compensation Insurance: A Primer for Public Health

David F. Utterback,
Alysha R. Meyers,
Steven J. Wurzelbacher

Department of Health and Human Services
Centers for Disease Control and Prevention
National Institute for Occupational Safety and Health

January 2014

This document is in the public domain and may be freely copied or reprinted.

Disclaimer

Mention of any company or product does not constitute endorsement by the National Institute for Occupational Safety and Health (NIOSH). In addition, citations to Web sites external to NIOSH do not constitute NIOSH endorsement of the sponsoring organizations or their programs or products. Furthermore, NIOSH is not responsible for the content of these Web sites. All Web addresses referenced in this document were accessible as of the publication date.

Ordering Information

To receive documents or other information about occupational safety and health topics, contact NIOSH:
Telephone: 1–800–CDC-INFO (1–800–232–4636)
TTY: 1-888-232-6348
Email: cdcinfo@cdc.gov
Or visit the NIOSH Web site at www.cdc.gov/niosh

For a monthly update on news at NIOSH, subscribe to NIOSH eNews by visiting www.cdc.gov/niosh/eNews.

DHHS (NIOSH) Publication No. 2014–110
January 2014

SAFER • HEALTHIER • PEOPLE™

Foreword

Occupational safety and health research and surveillance are essential for the prevention and control of injuries, illnesses and hazards that arise from the workplace. Research and surveillance can fill gaps in knowledge about where hazards exist and what interventions are effective at preventing workplace injuries, illnesses and fatalities. Workers' compensation insurance records are a resource used for these primary prevention purposes. In addition, workers' compensation records may be used for early detection of health outcomes in populations of workers which is part of secondary prevention. They may also be used to help identify effective medical treatment which is part of tertiary prevention.

Workers' compensation insurance covers nearly all workers in the U.S. and provides those who are injured or become ill as a result of work with medical treatment, a portion of lost wages, and a lump sum for some permanent impairments. Nonetheless, there are limitations to conducting studies that rely on workers' compensation records since not all injuries and illnesses result in claims being filed. Furthermore, the data that are collected are not readily combined if obtained from multiple sources since requirements vary substantially among the states.

The National Institute for Occupational Safety and Health (NIOSH) joined with a number of public and private sector co-sponsors to convene two workshops on the use of workers' compensation data for occupational safety and health. Creation of this document was suggested at the second workshop as a means to describe elements of the workers' compensation insurance programs in the U.S. and the potential to utilize the records for public health purposes.

Public health agencies, the workers' compensation industry, trade associations and the state-level programs share interests in utilizing these data to protect workers from occupational injuries and illnesses. To help facilitate these goals, NIOSH has created a Center for Workers' Compensation Studies. Further information on the center may be obtained at http://www.cdc.gov/niosh/topics/workerComp/CWCS/.

John Howard, M.D.
Director
National Institute for Occupational Safety and Health
Centers for Disease Control and Prevention

Acknowledgements

We thank the participants at the Use of Workers' Compensation Data for Occupational Safety and Health Workshop that was held in Washington, DC in June 2012 for suggesting that a document like this primer be developed. Many of those participants and other stakeholders provided essential input on the scope and contents of this primer. We also thank the internal and external reviewers for their valuable comments.

Acronyms and Abbreviations

AASCIF – American Association of State Compensation Insurance Funds
ACORD – Association for Cooperative Operations Research and Development
ACS – American Community Survey
AIA – American Insurance Association
CBP – County Business Patterns
CDC – Centers for Disease Control and Prevention
CES – Current Employment Statistics
CFOI – Census of Fatal Occupational Injuries
CFR – Code of Federal Regulations
CPS – Current Population Survey
DHHS – Department of Health and Human Services
EDI – Electronic Data Interchange
FEIN – Federal Employer Identification Number
FROI – First Report of Injury
FTE – Full-time Equivalent
HIPAA – Health Insurance Portability and Accountability Act
IAIABC – International Association of Industrial Accident Boards and Commissions
ICD – International Classification of Disease
IRS – Internal Revenue Service
MSHA – Mine Safety and Health Administration
NAICS – North American Industry Classification System
NASI – National Academy of Social Insurance
NAIC – National Association of Insurance Commissioners
NCOIL – National Conference of Insurance Legislators
NCCI – National Council on Compensation Insurance
NIOSH – National Institute for Occupational Safety and Health
OES – Occupational Employment Statistics
OIICS – Occupational Injury and Illness Classification System
OSHA – Occupational Safety and Health Administration
PCIAA – Property and Casualty Insurers Association of America
PEO – Professional Employment Organizations
QCEW – Quarterly Census of Employment and Wages
SDS – Supplementary Data System
SIC – Standard Industrial Classification System
SOC – Standard Occupational Classification System
SOII – Survey of Occupational Injuries and Illnesses
TPA – Third-party Administrator
WCIO – Workers' Compensation Insurance Organizations
WCRI – Workers' Compensation Research Institute

Table of Contents

Foreword iii

Acknowledgements iv

Acronyms and Abbreviations iv

1. Introduction 1

2. Background 2

3. Brief History of Workers' Compensation in the U.S. 4

4. Workers' Compensation Insurance Benefits 7

5. Workers' Compensation Insurance Providers 11

6. State Workers' Compensation Agencies 12

7. Third-Party Administrators 13

8. Types of Policies 13

9. Policy Premiums 18

10 Workers' Compensation Records 19

11. Standardized Codes and Systems in Workers' Compensation 21

12. Loss Prevention 22

13. Workers' Compensation Associations 23

14. Public Health Research and Surveillance 25

15. Public Health Regulations 26

16. Breaking through Barriers 27

References 29

Tables

Table 1 8

Table 2 14

Table 3 16

Appendices

Appendix A: Workers' Compensation Primer Glossary 35

Appendix B: Preparing for Engagement 41

1. Introduction

The purpose of this document is to help public health researchers and practitioners, particularly those in occupational safety and health, to broaden their understanding of workers' compensation insurance, relevant aspects of the insurance industry records, and the potential uses of that information for public health purposes. Workers' compensation insurance has been established in all states to provide income protection, medical treatment, and rehabilitation for employees who are injured or become ill as a result of work. Workers' compensation claims and medical treatment records along with other information resources have been used to conduct occupational safety and health research and surveillance and to identify intervention needs.

> Two workshops on the use of workers' compensation data for public health purposes have been held and proceedings are available.

Several government agencies and private organizations sponsored two workshops in September 2009 and June 2012 on the use of workers' compensation data for occupational safety and health purposes. The workshops featured discussions of opportunities for collaboration in the analysis of workers' compensation data in order to help reduce the risks of occupational injuries and illnesses. Participants included representatives from private insurance carriers, insurance associations, self-insured corporations, academic institutions and government agencies.

Presentations in the first workshop described differences among state laws, proper interpretation of common industry terms, proprietary interests in insurance data, public release of internal analyses, methods for linking workers' compensation records with other health and employment records, and independent analysis of claims data by health scientists, economists and government agencies [NIOSH 2010; Utterback et al. 2012]. One of the principal messages from the first workshop was that even though workers' compensation records are primarily designed and used by the insurance industry to administer claims, public health investigators are interested in them for prevention and control of occupational injuries and illnesses. The interested parties have different perspectives on the value and potential uses of workers' compensation data. Relationships would need to build trust and respect for the various stakeholder perspectives to foster collaboration.

The second workshop included discussions of six draft white papers along with 35 platform and poster presentations on research with workers' compensation data [NIOSH 2013a]. Although much progress is being made in understanding the merits of workers' compensation data resources, significant limitations exist. For example, these data appear to constitute an incomplete record of occupational injuries and illnesses at the state level. While standards for collecting and compiling the data exist, they are not universally used. Some fields on the record forms are often blank or incomplete and essential information for public health purposes, such as occupation, race, ethnicity, and duration of employment, may not be recorded. Multiple parties add data to the records at various stages as claims work their ways through the employees, employers, medical facilities, third-party administrators and state agencies. Nonetheless, important public health research can be conducted with available data as long as the limitations and their effects on generalizability are considered.

At the end of the second workshop, some commented that the public health and the insurance communities may have different interpretations of terms in common usage and overcoming that barrier might be facilitated by a summary of the workers' compensation industry and a crosswalk of terminology used by each group. A team began work on this document as a result.

Following the background and brief history of the workers' compensation programs in the U.S., this primer describes: (1) benefits and premiums; (2) the relationship between premiums and safety incentives; (3) roles of insurers, state agencies and third party administrators; (4) types of policies;

(5) claims and other workers' compensation insurance information on medical treatments, costs and disability status; (6) limitations of current industry data standards; (7) loss prevention programs; and (8) public health research, surveillance and regulations. A glossary of workers' compensation terms begins on page 35 and a guide for prospective research and surveillance projects follows on page 41.

2. Background

The economic and social burden of occupational injuries and illnesses can only be roughly estimated [Leigh and Marcin 2012; Leigh 2011]. Uncertainties are due to many factors including: (1) workers receive only a portion of regular wages through workers' compensation; (2) occupational illnesses are frequently not compensated; (3) medical treatment costs for many occupational injuries are paid by other insurance; (4) insurance data are fragmented; and (5) data are protected for proprietary and personal identification purposes. No central repository for workers' compensation claims information exists in the U.S.

> Workers' compensation data are likely to be more complete for acute injuries and more representative of population risks than occupational illness data.

The National Academy of Social Insurance (NASI), a non-governmental organization, produces an annual report on workers' compensation insurance. The most recent version, Workers' Compensation Benefits, Coverage, and Costs, 2010, states that workers' compensation insurance covered more than 124 million U.S. workers at a total estimated cost to employers of $71 billion in 2010 [Sengupta et al. 2012]. Total insured medical payments to providers and insured cash benefits to workers were estimated at $28.1 billion and $29.5 billion, respectively.

Most workers' compensation insurance carriers are private entities except for exclusive state insurance funds in North Dakota, Ohio, Washington and Wyoming. Also, twenty states offer state-sponsored nonprofit competitive insurance companies or state licensed mutual insurance plans, some to only selected portions of the market such as those employers that are unable to obtain insurance coverage in the voluntary market. There are typically dozens if not hundreds of private carriers in each state. Large employers in the U.S. are often self-insured under rules established by the states.

Workers' Compensation Records

Workers' compensation insurance, in various forms, covers in excess of 90% of the U.S. wage and salary workers [Sengupta et al. 2012]. Ideally, each workplace injury or illness requiring medical care covered by workers' compensation would result in a record being created for the claim. The primary purpose for the record is to ensure proper payment to injured or ill workers and to the medical providers. Yet the record may contain useful information for public health purposes on the nature of the injury or disorder, the part-of-body, the event or exposure, industry sector, occupation, and the worker's ability to continue working or disability status. Descriptive contents may provide additional information on materials related to the event such as biological, chemical, ergonomic or physical hazards.

Medical records for workers' compensation cases can provide further information about the extent and severity of the injury plus information about the injured workers such as gender, age, race/ethnicity, and other chronic health conditions that may exacerbate an injury. Workers' compensation medical records also identify disabilities that result from the occupational injuries or illnesses and billing records can contain information on treatments and costs for the medical portion of the claims.

Insurance carriers and self-insured entities are required to provide state government agencies with claims information that is used for administrative requirements such as oversight and to conduct hearings for adjudication of disputes. The level of detail and quality of information vary among the data providers. Nonetheless, in each state, a government agency has longitudinal data that may be suitable for public health research and surveillance purposes. It is noteworthy that the Health Insurance Portability and Accountability Act (HIPAA) Privacy Rule exempts workers' compensation medical information from its disclosure restrictions.[1]

If information from multiple sources or jurisdictions could be combined, workers' compensation insurance records would permit better analysis and tracking of occupational injuries and some diseases. In public health, use of these tracking systems is called surveillance. (See box for a definition.) Health scientists, economists, and others use large surveillance data sets for informative analyses of trends in incidence and costs, identification of health hazards associated with new technologies, evaluation of injury and illness prevention program effectiveness, and to provide employers with information needed to protect their workforce.

> The U.S. Centers for Disease Control and Prevention (CDC) defines public health surveillance as the "ongoing systematic collection, analysis, and interpretation of health data essential to the planning, implementation, and evaluation of public health practices, closely integrated with the timely dissemination of these data to those who need to know."

Limitations on Records Utility

For public health research and surveillance purposes, workers' compensation data are likely to be more representative of population risks for acute injuries than they are for occupational illnesses. Some investigators have used limited workers' compensation data to estimate the frequency, magnitude, severity, and cost of compensated injuries and to examine trends over time. Several papers at the 2012 workshop described deficiencies in workers' compensation records for injury and illness surveillance purposes, even for more severe injuries such as amputations, fractures and concussions [NIOSH 2013a].

Combining workers' compensation data from a number of jurisdictions is a major technical challenge. Each state legislature and the District of Columbia establish workers' compensation requirements[2] with significant variations. For example, states vary in the coverage of compensable cumulative injuries such as carpal tunnel syndrome, levels of payments for partial and total disability, both temporary and permanent, and the minimum number of days away from work to qualify for wage-replacement compensation. In many states, employers with small numbers of employees, temporary employees and other groups, such as farm employees, are excluded from coverage requirements. Certain groups of workers such as railroad, longshore, many maritime and all Federal employees are covered by rules established at the national level. Special compensation funds have been established at the Federal level for atomic weapons workers and for those disabled by black lung disease.

Another factor that makes it difficult to combine data from multiple sources is the lack of national data standards. For example, although some nationally standardized data coding systems are available, such as Occupational Injury and Illnesses Classification System (OIICS), and North American Industry Classification System (NAICS), they are not universally used across the states. In fact, workers' compensation rate-making bodies like the National Council on Compensation Insurance (NCCI) and several state rating bureaus use coding systems that pre-date OIICS and NAICS systems. These coding systems are discussed in subsequent chapters.

---

[1] More on the exclusion of workers' compensation medical records from the HIPAA Privacy Rule can be found at http://www.hhs.gov/ocr/privacy/hipaa/understanding/coveredentities/workerscomp.html
[2] This document uses "requirements" as a substitute term for legislation, statutes, rules and regulations since the sources for the legal obligations vary among the states.

Furthermore, access to workers' compensation data can be difficult to obtain. Insurance carriers are usually private businesses that manage very large data sets in integrated, proprietary systems. These data are generally not shared with external groups. Some insurance organizations like NCCI routinely collect standardized data from insurance carriers in many states but their contracts protect the proprietary interests of the contributing carriers and restrict data uses to issues directly related to estimating or recommending insurance premium rates for establishments within industries. Only one private insurance entity, The Liberty Mutual Research Institute for Safety, has published extensive peer-review articles related to injury and illness prevention based on workers' compensation records [Courtney 2010].

Even when conducting analyses of workers' compensation data from a single state, there are characteristics of the workers' compensation data that limit its utility. Multiple researchers have reported limitations on the utilization of workers' compensation for occupational injury and illness research and surveillance. Azaroff, et al. [2002] described a number of filters that limit the reporting and filing of cases and the subsequent development of a medical record or workers' compensation claim following a workplace injury or illness. Several investigators have reported much less than full participation in workers' compensation for occupational injuries and illnesses with up to half or more of the compensable claims going unreported [Biddle et al. 1998; Rosenman et al. 2000; Fan et al. 2006; Scherzer et al. 2008; Lipscomb et al. 2009].

> Each state has its own set of rules about which employers are required to obtain workers' compensation insurance.

Leigh [2012] estimated that only 21% of the total economic burden of occupational injuries and illnesses was paid by workers' compensation insurance carriers. Others describe the difficulty in estimating the portion of the burden that is shifted to other social and health insurance programs [Boden et al. 2001] such as when workers with occupational injuries and illnesses file disability claims with the Social Security Administration [O'Leary et al. 2012].

3. Brief History of Workers' Compensation in the US

Following European examples from the 19th century, states in the U.S. began to develop workers' compensation laws in the early 1900's to address the increasing risks of occupational injuries and illnesses associated with the industrial revolution. Initial laws in several states were declared unconstitutional but, in 1911, Wisconsin became the first state to establish a workers' compensation system that withstood constitutional challenges in the courts. By 1920, most states and territories[3] had followed suit. Mississippi was the last state to adopt a workers' compensation law in 1948.[4] These laws provide partial benefits to affected workers and protect employers from tort suits for occupational injuries and illnesses in nearly all cases. This "grand bargain" circumvents lengthy, expensive trials where the burden of proof was on the employee and removed a source of financial uncertainty for the employer.

Since the beginning of workers' compensation programs in the U.S., nearly all employers have

---

[3] References to state workers' compensation laws in this document should be read to include the territories of Guam and the Virgin Islands plus the District of Columbia, all of which have separate statutes and regulations.

[4] For greater details on the history and development of workers' compensation laws in Europe and the U.S., readers are directed to http://www.iaiabc.org/files/Resources/2006HistoryofIAIABC.pdf, http://eh.net/encyclopedia/workers-compensation/, http://www.ncbi.nlm.nih.gov/pmc/articles/PMC1888620/, or http://www.aascif.org/public/1.1.1_history.htm

been required to have insurance to cover payments for: (1) medical costs resulting from occupational injuries and some occupational illnesses suffered by workers; and (2) partial replacement of injured or ill workers' lost wages, also known as indemnity. Death benefits are paid to survivors for occupational fatalities. These benefits are paid only for claims where workers were injured or became ill due to conditions that "arise out of and in the course of employment," with restrictions that vary substantially among the 50 states due to legislation and case law. In return for this coverage, employers are granted immunity from employee law suits (tort litigation) for nearly all occupational injuries and illnesses. Thus workers' compensation insurance is structured to be the sole employee remedy for restitution subsequent to occupational injuries and illnesses. Some exceptions exist for willful injuries and gross negligence.

Mandatory Coverage
Each state has its own set of requirements about which employers are compelled to obtain workers' compensation insurance. Varying factors are generally the industry sector of the employer, the minimum number of employees, length of employment, and, in some cases, the familial relationship of the employee with the employer. The minimum number of employees requiring provision of workers' compensation coverage varies between one and five across the states. Some states exclude agricultural employers with less than a specified number of employees. Some states exclude self-employed workers while other states provide an option for their coverage. Some states exclude corporate officers in limited liability corporations without other employees. Other states have specific workers' compensation rules for industry sectors such as mining and construction. The employment relationships of employers with employees versus contractors are clearly defined in many states.[5]

Since the enactment of Texas workers' compensation legislation in 1913, employers in that state have been allowed to voluntarily participate in workers' compensation insurance coverage. Those employers who choose to opt out of coverage are not protected from tort suits by the injured or ill workers, or by surviving family members in case of fatalities. Any medical expenses are the responsibility of the injured or ill workers. No payments are required for the workers' lost earnings for the duration of their recovery period or for permanent disabilities. More recently, Oklahoma legislation that was enacted in May 2013 allows employers to opt out of workers' compensation insurance. In this state, employers who opt out are required to have an internal compensation program for occupational injuries and illnesses that is consistent with Employee Retirement Income Security Act (ERISA) [Oklahoma Insurance Department 2013].

Basis for Insurance Premiums
Throughout the history of workers' compensation in the U.S., premiums for insurance policies have been determined by a set of factors related to employer risks, primarily the mix of occupational classes they employ. Employers are assigned to work classifications[6] according to state-sanctioned rating bureau guidelines. In general, employers in classifications with greater injury and illness risks and loss costs have higher "manual rates." For example, a roofing contractor generally has a higher manual rate than a bank. Recommended or specified manual rates must be approved by the state regulators in most cases. Additionally, those employers which qualify for experience rating and that have a history of greater injury and illness claims and costs within the risk classes are charged even higher premiums through the application of an experience modification factor. Those employers with fewer claims and lower loss costs benefit from lower premiums.

---

[5]For greater details on workers' compensation trends and individual state requirements, readers are directed to the annual NASI report [Sengupta et al. 2012] and the annual report produced by the U.S. Chambers of Commerce [U.S. Chamber of Commerce 2012].
[6]The classifications do not directly correspond to Standard Industry Classification (SIC) or NAICS codes or occupational classification systems, such as the Standard Occupation Classes (SOC).

Motivations for Prevention

From the beginning of workers' compensation insurance laws in the U.S., the experience modification factor was intended to encourage employers to invest in safety. A history of elevated claims frequencies and costs results in higher insurance premiums for the employer. Adoption of effective safety strategies reduces occupational injuries and illnesses which should decrease future premiums. Additionally, many states have enacted legislation that requires carriers to provide premium discounts for the presence of employer-based leading indicators such as safety and health programs which meet specific criteria. Moreover, most carriers provide loss prevention services to client employers in order to limit escalation of claims costs and insurance premiums. Some states, for example Texas, Missouri and Arkansas, mandate that insurance carriers provide loss prevention services to clients and many specify that the services shall be provided at no additional cost beyond the annual premium.

> New types of workers' compensation insurance policies have been developed to cover the recent changes in the relationships between employees and employers.

Recent Changes in the Industry and Market

The workers' compensation insurance market is dynamic. Both the nature of work and workforce are changing. In recent years, the mix of industries and technologies in the U.S. have changed and the workforce is aging [Restrepo and Shuford 2011] and increasingly non-English speaking [Hakimzadeh and Cohn 2007] and obese [Ostbye et al. 2007; Trogden et al. 2007; Schmid et al. 2012]. In the past couple of decades, there have been substantial changes in state laws that affect workers' compensation policies and procedures. Workers' compensation insurance requirements on issues such as managed care organizations, limited physician choice, vocational rehabilitation, minimum standards of care, and restrictions on treatment options have been enacted in many states. Meanwhile, medical costs for claims have escalated [Shuford et al. 2009] and litigation of claims is common in many states [Willborn et al. 2012].

Changes in the relationships between employees and employers have created needs for newer workers' compensation insurance policy types. For example, contingent work arrangements through temporary employment agencies and professional employer organizations (PEO) are becoming more common [Smith et al. 2010]. These emergent work arrangements can complicate coverage and incentives for injury prevention. PEOs primarily have provided human resource and management services to client employers although they increasingly employ workers in other industries. PEOs result in co-employment by the host agency and the client employer. Newer workers' compensation policy arrangements have been developed for PEOs and similar employment leasing organizations [Shuford 2013] since a single host agency may employ workers at different times in industries with various risk classifications.

> The relationship between claims frequencies and costs and the employers' premium is intended to encourage investments to reduce the risk of injuries and illnesses.

In contrast, workers who are employees of a temporary agency are covered under the workers' compensation policy for that agency, not that of the client employer. Independent contractors, which are defined in the workers' compensation statutes in many states, are not covered by the policy of the contracting employer, e.g. the general contractor at a construction site. Also, independent contractors which are self-employed persons are qualified for workers' compensation insurance in some, but not all, states. Each of these arrangements can blur the responsibility for provision of workers' compensation coverage and has resulted in a lack of coverage for some workers.

Insurance Industry Resources

Many organizations produce information that is used by various parts of the workers' compensation insurance industry. The U.S. Department of Labor formerly compiled reports on benefits and costs and annual summaries of changes in state workers' compensation requirements. They also employed regional experts on workers' compensation. The federal efforts have shifted and some of the products have been replaced by private or nonprofit entities such as NASI and a number of others. For example, a biannual report that compares the average cost of workers' compensation insurance per $100 of employer payroll among states is published by the State of Oregon [Oregon Department of Consumer and Business Services 2012]. The roles and contributions of a number of these insurance organizations appears later in this document.

Effectiveness of State Laws
The comparative impact of the various state requirements has been a source of debate over the entire history of workers' compensation in the U.S. Federalization of the programs has been suggested from time to time. The Occupational Safety and Health Act in 1970 created the National Commission on State Workers' Compensation Laws which, after public meetings and comment period, proposed Federal minimum standards for state programs if the states did not substantially improve their laws. Related Congressional actions failed to pass. The Commission did develop a set of recommendations for the state programs.[7] Changes in state requirements subsequent to those recommendations have been periodically reviewed which indicate partial adoption by each of the states.[8]

According to national surveillance data, the frequency and rate of occupational injuries have declined over the past several decades [Sengupta et al. 2012; U.S. Bureau of Labor Statistics 2012]. In 2010, employer costs for workers' compensation benefits as a proportion of payroll were at the lowest level in 30 years [Sengupta et al. 2012]. There has also been a general trend across the states to limit compensation for disabled workers [Spieler and Burton 2012]. Whether the surveillance trends are due to reduced injuries, increases in underreporting, or other factors is the subject of ongoing research.

4. Workers' Compensation Insurance Benefits

Payments for workers' compensation claims can be for employee medical treatment, loss of wages (indemnity), vocational rehabilitation, permanent disability, and death. The rules for the level of payment vary tremendously among the states with a few exceptions. First, all medical expenses are the responsibility of the insurance provider without co-payment by the claimant but may be subject to legislated time limits and to medical fee schedules. These covered costs include the initial treatment and subsequent treatments plus physical therapy or vocational rehabilitations. Second, indemnity payments to the worker who misses work for greater than the minimum waiting period are provided tax-free. Third, most states provide wage replacement payments for the initial waiting period after lost work time exceeds a number of days that is set by the individual states (Table 1). For example, if the initial waiting period for indemnity payments is five calendar days, payments for that initial period would be made once the lost work time on that claim exceeds a separate minimum period such as 21 calendar days. This latter minimum time period is called the retroactive period.

> Payments for workers' compensation claims cover employee medical treatment, loss of wages, vocational rehabilitation, permanent disability and death.

---

[7] http://www.workerscompresources.com/National_Commission_Report/national_commission_report.htm
[8] http://www.ncbi.nlm.nih.gov/pubmed/15182746, http://www.ssa.gov/policy/docs/ssb/v65n4/v65n4p24.pdf http://www.workerscompresources.com/, National_Commission_Report/National_Commission/1-2004/Jan2004_nat_com.htm

Table 1. Waiting period for claimant to receive wage replacement benefits and the retroactive period which, if exceeded, results in payment for the waiting period

State	Waiting Period (days) [1]	Retroactive (days) [2]
AL	3	21
AK	3	28
AR	7	14
AZ	7	14
CA	3	14
CO	3	14
CT	3	14
DE	3	7
DC	3	14
FL	7	21
GA	7	21
HI	3	
ID	5	14
IL	3	14
IN	7	21
IA	3	14
KS	7	21
KY	7	14
LA	7	42
ME	7	14
MD	3	14
MA	5	21
MI	7	14
MN	3	10
MS	5	14
MO	3	14
MT	4	
NE	7	42
NV	5	6
NH	3	14
NJ	7	7
NM	7	28
NY	7	14
NC	7	21

Table 1. Waiting period for claimant to receive wage replacement benefits and the retroactive period which, if exceeded, results in payment for the waiting period (continued)

ND	5	5
OH	7	14
OK	3	
OR	3	14
PA	7	14
RI	3	
SC	7	14
SD	7	7
TN	7	14
TX	7	14
UT	3	14
VT	3	10
VA	7	21
WA	3	14
WV	3	7
WI	3	7
WY	3	9

[1] The minimum number of days away from work to qualify for indemnity payments, also known as the waiting period.

[2] If away from work for a number of days in excess of the retroactive period, claimant qualifies for indemnity payment for the waiting period.

Source: 2011 Chambers of Commerce Workers' Compensation Laws, Chart IX, (see caveats pp. 78 – 79 in reference)

Temporary Disabilities

Temporary and permanent disability benefits can be in the form of partial or total benefits. Temporary partial benefits would be merited when workers are away from work beyond the specified minimum period but able to return to work in a limited capacity that would partially affect their income. Temporary total disability benefits occur when the worker is unable to be employed in any capacity for a period of time that exceeds the specified waiting period. Many states have set time limits on temporary total disability indemnity payments such as 104 weeks. These benefits may convert to temporary partial benefits if the worker is able to return to work part-time for limited periods or if able to complete work in another position at a lower pay rate.

Permanent Disabilities

Permanent partial disability payments are awarded for workers who may no longer return to work with sufficient capacity to perform their prior duties or if they lose part or all of the function of a specific body part due to a work-related amputation or other disability. The loss of a body part or function is often compensated based on a fee schedule such that a set multiplier of the average wage is paid either as a lump sum or over a period of time. Many states also provide permanent partial coverage for disfigurement of the face or other body parts.

The extent of permanent partial disability is determined by the degree of impairment at the point of "maximal medical improvement" in order to settle the case. Impairment is usually determined according to medical references such as the American Medical Association Guides to the Evaluation of Permanent Impairment [Cocchiarella and Anderson 2001].

Permanent total disability indemnity payments are made to those workers who can no longer be employed in any capacity. Depending on the state, these payments may continue until retirement age, for the life of the individual, or until disability payments are received from another source such as the Social Security Administration.

In some cases, the portions of the disability that are attributed to work and non-work conditions can factor in the amount of the disability payment. For example, in some jurisdictions, a worker who is disabled as a result of occupational exposures to a respiratory hazard may have their benefits reduced if a non-occupational exposure, such as smoking, is demonstrated to have contributed to the impairment.

Death benefits are paid to survivors of the worker who was killed on the job. The level of benefits usually varies with the number of dependents. Although generally a function of the average weekly wage, death benefits are often limited by a minimum and maximum amount but may last for the lifetime of the surviving spouse or until dependent children attain 18 years of age or older in certain cases.

Settlement of Claims

Lump sum settlements, also known as negotiated settlements or compromise and release agreements, in lieu of limited periodic payments, have been increasing for disabilities covered by workers' compensation insurance. These agreements are reached between the disabled employee, the employer and the insurance provider. In some states, settlements may cover only indemnity portions of a claim, with future medical benefits provided, while others allow payouts for future medical care (including Medicare set-asides,[9] if appropriate). Often times, the settlements must be approved by a state workers' compensation authority.

> Future obligations on a claim are handled in the form of reserves that are established for open ended claims.

Claim Costs and Reserves

Claims that are not settled through mutual agreement remain open until all payments for medical treatments, rehabilitation and indemnity have been completed and the worker returns to work, reaches the maximum indemnity period or retirement age or dies. As a result, the cost of a claim can continue to grow. Future

---

[9]Medicaid set-asides for occupational injuries and illnesses are explained at http://www.medicare.gov/supplement-other-insurance/how-medicare-works-with-other-insurance/who-pays-first/workers-comp-payments.html.

obligations on a claim are handled in the form of reserves that are established for open ended claims and are dependent on the nature of the injury and the likelihood of the rehabilitation of the worker. Reserves typically represent estimates of the most likely future cost of the claim, which approximates the mode of the distribution of claims of that type, rather than the mean.

With the open-ended nature of longer duration claims, insurance carriers often value (estimate cost of) the claims based on the payments made to date, the payments plus reserves, or the payments plus reserves as of a certain period of time, such as 30 months after the date of injury. Claims can also be valued using "factor-adjusted" methods that calculate costs by applying actuarial loss development factors that attempt to estimate the ultimate payout amounts for the claims. For the "factor-adjusted" method, reserves therefore represent the mean future cost of claims of the same type. This method is applied to groups of claims and is used by insurance underwriters for analyzing aggregated claims for loss trends. A potential drawback with "factor-adjusted" methods is that their values are usually higher than the actual values of the individual claim (since the mean is always higher than the mode and median in claim cost distributions) [Wurzelbacher et al. 2013]. Some carriers use yet other cost valuation methods.

5. Workers' Compensation Insurance Providers

The workers' compensation insurance industry is complex with total per annum expenditures in excess of $70 billion [Sengupta et al. 2012]. The primary types of groups in the industry include insurance carriers, state regulatory agencies, third-party administrators and numerous trade organizations. Insurance providers may be privately-held corporations, mutual corporations (owned by the policy holders), and state or Federal agencies. All states except North Dakota permit self-insurance for qualified employers [U.S. Chamber of Commerce 2012].

Insurance Providers and Policies
The insurance providers are regulated by individual state requirements. Even nationwide insurance carriers must follow the requirements in each of the states where they offer coverage. In most states, private insurance carriers compete in the regulated voluntary market. Twenty states offer alternatives to the private insurers in the form of non-profit state-sponsored insurance programs. In addition, state funds are the exclusive providers of workers' compensation insurance in four states – North Dakota, Ohio, Washington and Wyoming.

Insurance providers employ a range of specialists such as actuaries, adjusters, underwriters, claims administrators and loss control consultants (see glossary). Brokers directly market insurance policies to employers and they may offer policies from a single insurance carrier or multiple competing carriers. Many private insurance providers specialize in specific industry sectors in which they are most familiar with risks. Large national carriers offer insurance across diverse sectors but may still focus on certain industries. Many private insurance providers also offer other lines of coverage beyond workers' compensation, such as property and liability.

Insurance providers typically issue annual policies. An employer may opt to change insurance carrier on the anniversary of the policy except in states with exclusive funds. Annual policies add to the competitiveness of the market yet they reduce the investment commitment of a carrier to client employers. For example, carriers are not likely to invest in cost reduction strategies such as safety equipment if the recovery of the investment would take several years to materialize.

Residual Market
The residual market customarily consists of those employers that are unable to obtain insurance coverage in the voluntary market. The residual market usually serves newer employers without sufficient years of experience in workers' compensation, employers with poor claims experience

or employers in high-risk industries unable to obtain a policy to underwrite their potential losses. However, the residual market in some states may include employers that voluntarily participate when there are economic or services advantages. All 24 state-sponsored insurance programs provide coverage for their residual markets. A few of the state-sponsored government insurance programs provide insurance coverage only to the residual market. Some states require the private insurance companies in their markets to write proportionate coverage for the residual market employers in the form of assigned-risk pools. The Burton primer on workers' compensation provides additional details on the residual market and assigned-risk pools [Burton 2004].

> The residual market usually serves newer employers without sufficient experience in workers' compensation, employers with poor claims experience, or employers in high-risk industries unable to obtain a policy to underwrite their potential losses.

6. State Workers' Compensation Agencies

Each state has an agency that provides administrative services for workers' compensation, has adjudicatory responsibilities in cases of disputes, and/or develops regulations and rules for the workers' compensation system consistent with the intent of legislative mandates. Portions of the agencies may operate as commissions, bureaus, or departments. They may be affiliated with other levels of government in the states such as labor, industry, insurance or commerce.

Collection of Records

All states require that some portion of the workers' compensation claims records be reported to the agency by employers (Table 2). In some cases only indemnity claims are reported yet in others all claims (including medical only claims) are reported. More and more states have developed automatic Web (internet)-based or telemetric reporting systems that use standard forms and require the use of standardized codes for fields in the forms. For example, the Workers' Compensation Insurance Organization (WCIO) part-of-body, nature of injury or illness, and cause of incident codes are used in nearly all jurisdictions.

> All states workers' compensation agencies require that some portion of the claims records be reported.

> HIPPA Privacy Rule exempts workers' compensation medical information from its disclosure restrictions. (See footnote 1)

State agencies may be restricted by requirements in the portions of the workers' compensation records which may be released to the public. In some states, those restrictions can extend to other in-state agencies as well. It bears repeating that HIPAA Privacy Rule exempts workers' compensation medical information from its disclosure restrictions.

Other Roles of State Agencies

Many state agencies oversee special funds that provide benefits to injured or ill workers whose employer failed to obtain the legally required coverage. Most states also offer second injury funds which reimburse employers for certain claims paid to workers with pre-existing injuries. A few state agencies, e.g. Ohio and Washington, provide safety grants to offset some portion of an employer's expenses for installation of safety equipment. Grants in other states, e.g. Massachusetts and Oregon, are made to support development of injury prevention training programs (Table 3).

A few states have research components in their workers' compensation agencies. These components may track expenditures, evaluate the implications of proposed legal changes, or consider other aspects of policy options. Many states, e.g. Florida [Florida Division of Workers' Compensation 2011], develop annual reports for their agencies that reveal the number of cases in various categories such as indemnity, medical-only and disallowed claims as well as the number of claims that are contested by the employer or the insurance provider. The reports may also describe recent changes to the requirements and the status of claims that are open and those that are closed. Other data may be presented on the average cost of claims for various injury and illness types as well as the distribution of claims across industry segments.

> Third-party administrators (TPA) are insurance organizations other than the brokers, providers, associations and the state agencies.

Web (Internet) Services

Most state agencies provide diverse services and extensive information via Web sites. Available services include injury, illness and death claim forms for employees and employers and the means to report suspected fraud. Proof of insurance coverage by individual employers may be obtained in some states through their Web sites. The Web site information may describe the rights and responsibilities of employees, employers, insurance carriers, medical providers, and the state agency according to requirements in the state. Many states provide plain-language guides for employees and employers that explain claims processing and appeals. Ombudsmen in some states may be contacted through the Web sites to assist claimants.

Most state agencies also use Web sites to promote safe and healthful working conditions and to provide information on safety and health program aids that can be readily used by employers. Other information on participation in various programs associated with premium discounts or penalties is offered as well. Lists of insurance providers as well as consultants and third party administrators are available on many state sites. Training on the workers' compensation requirements is often made available through the Web sites. Links to state statutes and regulations are common.

7. Third-Party Administrators

Third-party administrators (TPA) are insurance organizations other than the brokers, providers, associations and the state agencies. TPAs provide a wide range of services. They often complete the actual claims forms and may be the direct payer of benefits to workers and to medical providers. They can be the intermediary that reports the claim information to the respective state agency and they provide analytical reports to their clients. Self-insured businesses often employ TPAs for a diverse range of claim and insurance services. TPAs may complete and otherwise process claim forms for the employer, pool or group including an initial determination of compensability. Complete risk management information systems are offered by some TPAs.

In addition, they can provide services such as medical case management, medical bill review, and programs for the injured employee to return-to-work. Some TPAs provide investigation, subrogation and legal services to their clients. Pharmacy benefit management and Medicare set-aside services are some of the later additions to the TPA offerings. Yet others may provide loss prevention services and health and safety training for employees and employers. TPAs may also provide clients with their required Occupational Safety and Health Administration (OSHA) logs for recordable injuries and illnesses.

> Increasing risk retention by the employer is accommodated by the following insurance or policy types: guaranteed cost, dividend, retrospective rating, deductible, and self-insurance.

8. Types of Policies

Workers' compensation insurance policies vary in many ways. The most straightforward policies cover the claims costs due to a worker injury or illness experienced by a single employer at a single business establishment, i.e. location. Some employers have multiple establishments for a single policy and the risk classification for the individual establishments may be different, e.g. a manufacturer that also has a retail outlet. Yet other policies may cover workers at multiple establishments that change over time

Table 2. Required employer reporting of injuries, illnesses and deaths to State Workers' Compensation Bureaus.

State	Medical Treatment beyond 1st Aid Provided[1]	Indemnity Only (Min. No. Days)[2,3]
AL		Y(3)
AK	Y	
AR	Y	
AZ	Y	
CA		Y(1)
CO		Y(3)
CT		Y(1)
DE	Y	
DC	Y	
FL	Y	
GA		Y(7)
HI	Y	
ID	Y	Y(1)[4]
IL		Y(3)
IN		Y(1)
IA		Y(3)
KS		Y(1)
KY		Y(1)
LA		Y(7)
ME		Y(1)
MD		Y(3)
MA		Y(5)
MI		Y(7)
MN		Y(3)
MS		Y(5)
MO	Y	
MT	Y	
NE	Y	
NV	Y	
NH	Y	
NJ	Y	
NM	Y	
NY		Y(1)
NC		Y(1)
ND	Y	

Table 2. Required employer reporting of injuries, illnesses and deaths to State Workers' Compensation Bureaus (continued).

OH		Y(7)
OK	Y	
OR		Y(3)
PA		Y(1)
RI	Y	Y(3) [4]
SC	>$500	Y(1) [4]
SD	Y	Y(7) [4]
TN	Y	
TX		Y(1)
UT	Y	
VT	Y	Y(1) [4]
VA	Y	
WA		Y(1)
WV	Y	
WI		Y(3)
WY	Y	

[1] If Y, employers are required to report all claims that result in medical treatment beyond first aid to the workers' compensation bureau. (In SC, all claims with >$500 in medical expenses must be reported.)

[2] Employers are required to report all claims for occupational injuries and illnesses for workers missing work for a period of time in excess of these values.

[3] All deaths due to occupational injuries or illnesses must also be reported in all states.

[4] Additional reporting required for disabilities in excess of the number of days indicated.

Source: 2011 Chambers of Commerce Workers' Compensation Laws, Chart IX, (see caveats pp. 78 – 79 in reference)

Table 3. States with statutes, rules and/or regulations about employer-based occupational safety and health program elements plus states with approved state OSHA Plans or consultation programs only, 2011

State OS&H Regulations	States
Requirements	
Employer Written Safety and Health Program	CA[1], HI[2], LA[3], MN[4], NE, NV[5], NH[5], NC[6], WA
Employer/Employee Safety and Health Committee	AL[7], CA[4], CT[8], MN[9], MT[10], NE, NV[11], NH[10], NC[12], OR[13], TN[14], WA[5]
Insurer to Provide Loss Prevention Services	AR, CA, KS, MS, MO, MT, NM, OR, PA, RI, SD, TX
On-Site Inspection by Loss Prevention Services	AR[15], CA[16], DE[17], NM[18], NY[19], RI[20], TX[21]
Incentives	
Premium Reduction for Safety Program Elements	CO, DE[22], FL, HI, ME, NH, NM, NY, ND, OH, OK, PA, SD[23], UT[24], WI, WY[25]
Employer Penalty for Violation of Rule at Time of Injury	CA, IL, MA, MO, NC, WI
Safety Grant	MA[26], MN, NY, ND, OH, OR[26], UT, WA
Registry of S&H Practitioners	HI, LA, MO
State OSHA Plan	AK, AZ, CA, CT[27], HI, IL[27], IN, IA, KY, MD, MI, MN, NV, NJ[27], NM, NY[27], NC, OR, SC, TN, UT, VT, VA, WA, WY
State Consultation Program Only	AL, AR, CO, DE, FL, GA, ID, KS, LA, ME, MA, MS, MO, MT, NE, NH, ND, OH, OK, PA, RI, SD, TX, WV, WI

Information in this table was obtained from Web sites of state legislatures and agencies. Due to the difficulty in locating statutes, rules, regulations and relevant case law, some information may have been omitted from the table. Further information may be obtained from the primary author.

[1]Reduced documentation requirements if <10 employees; <20 employees and not on high hazard list and experience modification is <1.1; or < 20 employees and on designated low-hazard list.
[2]If >24 employees
[3]If > 15 employees
[4]For high hazard industries on list
[5]If >10 employees

[6] If experience modification factor is >1.5
[7] Upon written request of an employee
[8] If >25 employees or injury and illness rate greater than average for industry
[9] If > 25 employees or if in top 10% within industry lost-days rate or if top 25% of pure premium for all classes
[10] If >5 employees
[11] If >25 employees
[12] If >10 employees and experience modification factor >1.5
[13] Routine safety meetings also allowed
[14] If experience modification factor is >1.2
[15] Or other appropriate services if premium > $25,000, or if > $5,000 and loss ratio > 100%, or if loss ratio > 150%
[16] For targeted high hazard employers
[17] Fee is charged and employer required to participate in Workplace Safety Program discount
[18] If premium > $5,000, self-inspection is allowed
[19] If payroll > $800,000 and experience modification factor >1.2
[20] If premium > $25,000 and requested by employer
[21] If premium > $25,000 and loss ratio >1.0, or if premium > $5,000 and loss ratio > 2.5
[22] If premium > $3,161
[23] Unspecified penalty for establishments where deficiency has not been corrected at time of subsequent safety review
[24] If experience modification factor >1.0 or if 3-year loss ratio > 100% and if "work place safety program" not adopted after request from the insurer then 5% premium surcharge is allowed
[25] Based on reduced loss ratio attainment
[26] Grants available for training only
[27] Public sector employees only are covered by the state plan along with consultation program for most private businesses

such as one for a company in the residential construction industry.

If employees of the business routinely travel to other states, provisions that cover losses in the other states may be added to policies. If the business has employees located in multiple states, multiple policies are typically required. With workers' compensation records alone, it may be difficult to associate an injury or illness with an establishment when the policy covers multiple establishments.

In many states, employers are allowed to form groups or pools to obtain insurance in the voluntary markets or to combine as a self-insured entity. Membership in a group is usually restricted to similar industries. Other insurance arrangements include carve-outs, which are labor/management agreements,[10] and captives, i.e. an insurance company that is wholly-owned by a single employer or a group of employers and provides insurance to the owners' businesses.

Risk Retention

Workers' compensation insurance policies determine the amount of risk the employer retains for workplace injuries and illnesses. Risk retention may increase employer interest in reducing potential losses through safety and health prevention since they could be responsible for payments on some claims. In order of increasing risk retention by the employer are the following insurance or policy types: guaranteed cost, dividend, retrospective rating, deductible, and self-insurance [Thamann and Reitz 2000]. For example, with a guaranteed cost policy, the loss to the employer in a given policy year can never be more than the policy premium. On the other hand, with large deductible policies, the employer is self-insured up to an amount of the deductible yet obtains an insurance policy for excess coverage purchased from a provider. The deductible amounts may be per claim and/or aggregate and range from a few thousands of dollars to $1 million or more. Nonetheless, the carrier of the excess coverage is, according to the state regulators, responsible for the entire claim amount. The carrier then obtains reimbursement from the client employer through an agreed mechanism.

Self-insurance is a form of insurance that is generally limited to larger employers which demonstrate to their state workers' compensation regulating agency that they have the financial resources to make the equivalent of indemnity, medical and death benefit payments to their employees who suffer occupational injuries and illnesses. Qualifications for self-insurance vary among the states. For example, some require surety bonds. In Ohio, an exclusive state program, self-insurance is permitted only for those employers with a minimum of 500 employees.

Other Policies

As mentioned earlier, state-sponsored programs also provide insurance coverage for workers whose employer failed to obtain the required insurance policy. Most states also provide special coverage for second injuries which reduces the financial disincentives of employing a worker with an existing disability.

9. Policy Premiums

Premiums for workers' compensation insurance policies are determined by the risk classification of the insured employer, the size of the payroll, and in many cases, on the employer's past claims experience. "Manual rates" or "base rates" are set for each of the industry risk classes by actuarial organizations like NCCI and are expressed as the cost of insurance per $100 in payroll. The manual rate is then adjusted using an experience modification factor for those employers who are sufficiently large to be rated based on their claims history. The premium setting process and related terms are more fully explained in other sources such as A Primer on Workers' Compensation by John F. Burton, Jr.[11]

---

[10] "Carve out" has different meanings across the insurance industry. The definition used for workers' compensation insurance carve outs in California may be found at http://www.dir.ca.gov/dwc/carveout.html.

[11] Burton's Workers' Compensation Resource provides access to a wide range of relevant materials. http://workerscompresources.com/wp-content/uploads/2012/11/ND04A.pdf

Experience Modification Factor

In general, an employer's history of increasing numbers of claims and costs leads to higher experience ratings and higher overall premiums. The experience modification factor is usually affected more by the frequency of claims from the policy holder than by the total cost, although these rules vary among the states. The loss ratio is one of the factors used to calculate premiums and it is equal to the total costs for losses divided by total premiums paid. The loss ratio may be calculated for a single client, a risk class or for the insurance industry as a whole.

Other Premium Adjustments

The premium may be further altered by discounts that are awarded for multiple reasons. For example, discounts may encourage certain activities such as an employer's participation in a safety council, having joint labor management health and safety committees, or having documented safety and health programs. Some provide premium discounts for firms with drug and alcohol programs. Many mutual insurance companies provide dividends that effectively reduce the premiums.

10. Workers' Compensation Records

Workers' compensation claims records contain information that may be used to determine the frequency of injuries and illnesses plus indicators of morbidity severity such as medical treatments, their costs, hospitalizations, days away from work, types and percentages of disabilities, and rehabilitation. As mandated by the individual state laws, parts of workers' compensation records and record systems may be completed by employees, employers, medical providers, insurance carriers, third-party administrators, and the state agencies.

> Premiums for workers' compensation insurance policies are dependent on the risk classification of the employer, the size of the payroll, and in many cases, on the establishment's past claims experience.

> Not only can workers' compensation records be used to determine the frequency of injuries and illnesses, but also disability status, medical treatments, their costs, hospitalizations, days away from work, and rehabilitation.

The most common types of records are the claims forms for injury and illness and these are required in all states.

Yet other potentially useful records may be collected and retained by the carrier. These additional records may describe employer safety and health programs, work-site inspections and other loss prevention activities. Records may also exist on the current insurance status of individual employers, carrier enrollments to conduct business in the state, registrations of consultants and third-party administrators, adjudications and appeals, and self-insurance applications, among others. Access to these records may be restricted by the applicable laws in each state. Individual investigators need to verify all legal restrictions in each state of interest.

Standard Records

The most common claims record is the first report of injury (FROI) form. The form collects some demographic information on the injured or ill employee, disability status, and contact information for the employer, insurance carrier, and medical provider. Many states use the standard FROI developed through the Electronic Data Interchange (EDI) by the International Association of Industrial Accident Boards and Commissions (IAIABC). An example of the EDI form and instructions can be accessed at the Missouri Department of Labor and Industrial Relations Web site.[12] Three versions of this form are now in use across the participating states. Forms used by yet other states contain similar information but the range of forms is too broad to list each one of them.

---

[12] One example of an EDI FROI can be found at http://labor.mo.gov/DWC/Forms/WC-1-EDI-AI.pdf.

The EDI forms include sections on employee wage, gender, date of birth and date of hire, occupation, employment status, and number of dependents. The event fields include date, time of day, date employer was notified and date disability began, type of injury and affected body part, and descriptive information on the equipment involved, worker activities, work process, sequence of events, and check boxes for use of personal protective equipment. Dates for return to work or for deaths are also listed on the form. The medical treatment provider is also identified and their address is listed along with a checklist for the level of treatment (from none to hospitalization), and future lost work time anticipated. Many of the fields on the FROI use standard codes which are described below in section 11.

> The initiator of workers' compensation claims has a major role in ensuring that all fields in the FROI form are accurately completed. The initiator may be the employer, injured employee, insurance broker, TPA, or a treating physician depending on the state.

Subsequent reports of injury (SROI) for each claim may be completed at the time treatment is provided by a health care practitioner, when a benefit type is changed (e.g. from temporary total to permanent total disability), or when the claimant returns to work or dies. Thus, a series of reports may be available for each claim. A computerized record is generally used to combine the information from the claims record series.

Billing forms from treatment providers are another set of records that provide important information. These forms list the treatment costs and may include information on diagnosis and treatments (such as Current Procedural Terminology codes) which may differ from the FROI and SROI. The differences may result from additional medical testing or from aggravation of an existing condition such as an infection. Any changes in diagnosis should be recorded in the injury claim record system.

Another record system widely used in the U.S. is the Unit Statistical Report that is provided by insurers to NCCI and other workers compensation data collection organizations. These reports are initially valued at 18 months after policy effective dates and include premium and loss information on a state basis. Open claims are valued and reported annually for up to 10 years to track loss development.[13,14]

Limitations of Record Information

It is important to mention, once again, that the primary purpose for the injury and billing records is the timely payment of the injured or ill workers and their medical providers. Therefore, information in these records that is used for these purposes is likely to be more robust than other fields in the record systems. For example, diagnostic and treatment codes are more likely to be accurate and complete than information on occupation and employment status, particularly for medical only claims. An estimated 80% of all claims are medical only [Sengupta et al. 2012]. The statutory days away from work time limits for "medical only" versus "lost time" claims vary significantly from one state to another (Table 2).

> Information in the workers' compensation records that is used for payment of workers and medical providers is likely to be more accurate and complete than other fields in the record systems.

---

[13] set of slides that explain unit reporting is available at http://www.ncci.com/documents/DRW-2008-Unit-Data-Reporting.pdf

[14] NCCI's Statistical Plan for Workers Compensation and Employers Liability is applicable in Alaska, Alabama, Arizona, Arkansas, Colorado, Connecticut, District of Columbia, Florida, Georgia, Hawaii, Idaho, Illinois, Indiana, Iowa, Kansas, Kentucky, Louisiana, Maine, Maryland, Mississippi, Missouri, Montana, Nebraska, Nevada, New Hampshire, New Mexico, Oklahoma, Oregon, Rhode Island, South Carolina, South Dakota, Tennessee, Utah, Vermont, Virginia and West Virginia.

The information in many claim records evolves over time and delays in availability are to be expected. Statutes of limitation are common for workers filing claims for an occupational injury or illness and often extend to 2 years in many states. Employers are required to report claims information to state agencies within specified periods that vary among states – usually less than 15 days (Table 2). Employers and insurers are also required to maintain claims records for time periods that vary among the states. Records maintenance is one of the primary services provided to employers by TPAs.

Many of the terms used in the workers' compensation industry have specific meanings. For example, the term "claim," itself is subject to confusion as it is applied to the notification of the supervisor, notification of the insurer at the time of injury, the "first report" for the state workers' compensation agency, or a request for arbitration on the part of the worker. Some of these terms are defined in the glossary (p. 35). For any set of electronic data, it is important to obtain the applicable data dictionary that specifically defines each data element and each code used. An historical dictionary may be essential for longitudinal data. Additional limitations on claims information are described in the Background section of this document.

Disallowed and Zero-Cost Claims

Claims can be disallowed by insurance carriers or contested by the employer. The basis for denial is usually related to the degree of disability or the requirement that the injury or illness "arise out of and in the course of employment." Disallowed claims may be appealed to administrative or judicial bodies depending on the state and may result in litigation which follows established procedures in each jurisdiction.

Zero-cost claims may also occur but these are not the same as disallowed claims. The claim may have been initiated yet the injury or illness did not result in medical treatment or in lost work time. At least one state, Ohio, allows employers to pay the initial treatment and/or indemnity cost up to specified limits. If the claim is paid by the employer and remains within those limits, the claims records would indicate zero costs to the agency.

11. Standardized Codes and Systems in Workers' Compensation

Numerous standardized data coding systems are utilized for workers' compensation claims information. Some of these were specifically developed and adopted within the workers' compensation industry while other coding systems such as NAICS and International Classification of Disease (ICD) were developed for other purposes.

Standard Systems

There have been and are many attempts to standardize data for workers' compensation records. For example, WCIO led a collaborative effort to standardize codes for the part-of-body, nature of injury, and cause of event that are used across the workers' compensation insurance industry including NCCI, IAIABC and the Association for Cooperative Operations Research and Development (ACORD) but not in all jurisdictions. NCCI coding systems for industry risk classifications and a number of other factors are used in about 40 jurisdictions. IAIABC in collaboration with a number of states developed standardized forms that utilize several different data coding structures. The standards and codes have changed over time and different release versions have been adopted by states.[15] U.S. government coding systems are used extensively such as OIICS from the Bureau of Labor Statistics (BLS) and Federal Employer Identification Number (FEIN) from the Internal Revenue Service (IRS). The Standard Occupational Classification (SOC) and Standard Industry Classification (SIC) also continue to be used in some states.

Several states, e.g. California and New York, have developed their own codes for certain classes of workers' compensation information. Crosswalks may be available for some of the

---

[15] http://www.iaiabc.org/i4a/pages/index.cfm?pageid=3339

coding systems. Unfortunately, the comparisons are often uncertain. For example, it is not always possible to identify unique ICD codes for the NCCI injury classification codes and the OIICS nature of injury codes do not correspond one-to-one with WCIO recommended codes.

Portions of the individual records may be completed by parties unfamiliar with various coding systems which may lead to errors. For example, many employers may not know the codes for the nature of injury although online guides are available in many jurisdictions. Multi-source documents may be more prone to errors and omissions.

12. Loss Prevention

Many insurance carriers have loss prevention programs to identify and describe the particular risks that exist at policyholders' establishments, make recommendations for their abatement, and offer loss prevention[16] services to help policyholders manage these risks. They also assess risks that exist at establishments for which they contemplate underwriting new policies. For current policyholders, the primary purposes for the loss prevention services are to reduce the frequency and severity of workers' compensation claims and to improve the health and safety program of the client. Policyholders with higher premiums are more likely to receive routine loss prevention services from carriers than those with smaller premiums [Morin et al. 2013].

> In general, loss prevention programs identify and describe risks at policyholders' establishments and make recommendations for their abatement.

The provided services, which frequently are viewed as marketing tools to retain existing clients, may range from delivering relevant safety and health pamphlets and brochures to full risk characterizations that include recommendations for remediation with follow up inspections. Most small employers would not receive site visits unless their claims experience indicated a need for intervention.

Mandated Prevention Programs

All states have enacted legislation and developed related rules and regulations to reduce occupational injury and illness risks. The strategies employed by the states vary extensively and may include employer safety and health program requirements and incentives, insurance carrier loss prevention activities, registries of authorized occupational health and safety practitioners, and employer or organizational grants for risk mitigation and worker training (Table 3).[17] These inducements are often limited to those employers with greater than a minimum number of employees, minimum qualifying premiums, elevated experience modification factors, or that appear on lists of high hazard industries. Twelve states require workers' compensation insurance carriers to provide loss prevention services to many employers at no additional cost (Table 3). Requirement for these services is often limited to those policyholders with greater than a minimum number of employees, such as 25, or with premiums above minimum thresholds such as $25,000.

Carrier-based Loss Prevention Programs

Most large workers' compensation insurance carriers invest portions of their revenues in loss prevention programs [Dembe 1995; Nave and Veltri 2004; Ryan 2013] although the amounts or percentages are not readily available. According to one

---

[16] Note that "loss control" and "loss prevention" are terms that are often used interchangeably. In contrast, the term "loss reduction" is typically used to refer to the management of costs and disability once an injury or illness has occurred through programs such as case management and return-to-work.

[17] States that do not appear in Table 3 list of prevention requirements or incentives are Alaska, Arizona, Georgia, Idaho, Indiana, Iowa, Kentucky, Maryland, Michigan, New Jersey, South Carolina, Vermont, Virginia and West Virginia

recent report, 13% of large workers' compensation insurance clients, on average, receive loss control visits in a given year although that value varies widely by industry group (e.g. Manufacturing = 32%, Construction = 16%, Agriculture = 4%) [Ryan 2013]. For the most part, loss prevention programs collect information on hazards and other determinants of risks from employers either prior to the issuance of a policy, i.e. risk selection for underwriting, or as a means of providing services to existing clients. Depending on the size of the premium, loss prevention services may include conduct of site visits which frequently include walk-through inspections of facilities, interviews with employees, supervisors and managers, as well as reviews of the employer's safety and health program elements. The report for the initial survey is shared with the carrier's underwriting staff as well as a broker that may be involved in the transaction. These risk selection reports are considered privileged information and often only selected portions of the reports are shared with the client [Morin et al. 2013].

> The workers' compensation insurance industry is supported by many professional and trade associations that provide a range of services.

For new and existing clients, key elements of loss prevention reports, such as a description of the hazards identified and recommendations for their abatement, may be provided to the employer. The loss prevention staff may also communicate the need for improvements (such as specific training or documentation) to the employer's health and safety programs. They may also provide specific services such as training employees, supervisors and managers and make training materials and model program elements available. Industrial hygiene and ergonomic surveys are included as needed. Afterwards, the loss prevention program may track progress through follow-up communications with the employer. The loss prevention professional may assist the employer in the completion of a safety grant application if they are available.

Loss prevention records are not standardized except perhaps within insurance providers. The availability of mobile technology applications for loss prevention programs is increasing and may provide additional opportunities for data standards developments on hazards and employer health and safety program elements.

13. Workers' Compensation Associations and Organizations

The workers' compensation insurance industry is supported by a large number of professional and trade associations and other organizations that operate at the international, national, state and even local levels. Some are membership organizations that provide professional services such as annual meetings, education and training. Some are research organizations that complete work under contracts. Others are affiliations of state and provincial agency representatives. Only a few of the longest-standing organizations will be mentioned here.

Two of the oldest workers' compensation insurance industry associations are NCCI and IAIABC. These organizations date from the earliest state workers' compensation programs in the U.S.

According to their Web site, NCCI "is the largest provider of workers' compensation and employee injury data and statistics in the nation." NCCI receives proprietary claims information from insurance carriers in their member states in the form of a Unit Statistical Data report which guides setting of manual rates for their client jurisdictions. To support the reporting system, NCCI in conjunction with WCIO has developed a number of standard coding schemes for nature of injury, event causation, and part-of-body. In addition, NCCI standard codes for industry, occupation and other factors are used by the nearly 40 affiliate jurisdictions. NCCI also conducts research and other analyses across a range of issues in the workers' compensation insurance industry. Many of their reports may be accessed at https://www.ncci.com/nccimain/pages/default.aspx.

The IAIABC mission statement is "to improve the efficiency and effectiveness of workers' compensation systems throughout the world." Among its published strategic principles are: "provide a forum for regulators, stakeholders and experts to share information and discuss issues and solutions; assist jurisdictions in identifying opportunities for reducing costs and improving the delivery of benefits; and develop, analyze, and promulgate standards and uniform practices." IAIABC has published a number of important insurance industry documents and it sponsors and supports the EDI. Much of their information may be accessed at http://www.iaiabc.org/i4a/pages/index.cfm?pageid=3277.

Other workers' compensation organizations include WCRI whose mission statement is: "to be a catalyst for significant improvements in workers' compensation systems, providing the public with objective, credible, high-quality research on important public policy issues." The institute is an independent and not-for-profit organization providing peer-reviewed, objective information about workers' compensation systems. Most of their documents are available to members only but some useful information may be found at http://www.wcrinet.org/about.html.

According to the NASI Web site, the academy is a nonprofit, nonpartisan and non-governmental organization led by the nation's experts on social insurance. It evaluates programs and data to develop solutions to challenges on social insurance and economic security. NASI supports research and publishes documents on social insurance topics and produces an annual report on workers' compensation programs in the U.S. that may be obtained free of charge at http://www.nasi.org/about.

WCIO "is a voluntary association of statutorily authorized or licensed rating, advisory, or data service organizations that collect workers compensation insurance information in one or more states." Members of the WCIO are managers of boards and agencies within the jurisdictions. Its forum supports development of electronic data transmission standards for insurers and rating/advisory organizations. Additional information about WCIO and its range of products can be found at https://www.wcio.org/Document%20Library/AboutPage.aspx.

ACORD is an international organization that facilitates the development of open consensus data standards and standard forms for many segments of the insurance industry, and works with its members and partner organizations to drive implementation of those standards. Their information may be found at http://www.acord.org/Pages/default.aspx.

A couple of other organizations that are widely recognized in the insurance industry include: John F. Burton Jr.'s Workers' Compensation Resource which provides access to data, research, and other information pertaining to workers' compensation in the United States and other countries when possible. The resource offers open access to many publications such as the 1972 Report of the National Commission on State Workmen's Compensation Laws. The extensive workers' compensation information may be found at http://workerscompresources.com/. Dr. Burton also hosts an annual meeting for discussion of current workers' compensation research.

The Liberty Mutual Research Institute for Safety (LMRIS) is a research organization funded by a private insurance company. For over 60 years, the institute has conducted scientifically rigorous, peer-reviewed research to improve worker safety and health. They conduct laboratory and field studies and publish records-based research using workers' compensation data collected by Liberty Mutual Insurance. Extensive information on LMRIS can be found at http://www.libertymutualgroup.com/omapps/ContentServer?pagename=LMGroup/Views/LMG&ft=2&fid=1138356633468&ln=en

Other organizations that serve the workers' compensation insurance industry include the American Association of State Compensation Insurance Funds (AASCIF), American Insurance Association (AIA), National Association of Insurance Commissioners (NAIC), National Conference of Insurance Legislators (NCOIL), and Property and Casualty Insurers Association of America (PCIAA).

14. Public Health Research and Surveillance[18]

Public health is "the science and art of preventing disease, prolonging life and promoting health through the organized efforts and informed choices of society, organizations, public and private, communities and individuals" [Winslow 1920]. Fundamentally, public health relies on surveillance programs to describe the distribution of disease and injury, detect new and emerging diseases and disorders, target intervention activities to prevent their incidence, and monitor the effectiveness of those interventions. Workers' compensation records may be used for public health research and surveillance activities. The terms "research" and "surveillance" have specific meaning in Federal public health activities which are briefly discussed here.

Research

Federal regulations state that "research means a systematic investigation, including research development, testing and evaluation, designed to develop or contribute to generalizable knowledge" [45 Code of Regulations (CFR) 46.102(d)]. Investigators performing public health research or surveillance activities have the responsibility to ensure that the research is conducted in a manner consistent with legal and ethical requirements. All research involving human participants that is conducted or supported by the U.S. Department of Health and Human Services (DHHS) must comply with DHHS Policy for Protection of Human Research Subjects [45 CFR part 46]. Investigators should consult with their local institutional review board for assistance with development of research or surveillance projects to insure that human subjects are appropriately protected.

> Federal regulations state that "research means a systematic investigation, including research development, testing and evaluation, designed to develop or contribute to generalizable knowledge" (45 CFR 46.102(d)).

Surveillance

Public health surveillance is the systematic, ongoing collection, management, analysis, and interpretation of data followed by the dissemination of these data to public health programs to stimulate public health action [Thacker et al. 2012]. Surveillance systems can be used to monitor infectious and non-infectious diseases as well as injuries and deaths. Surveillance data can be primary in that they are collected for a specific public health purpose or they may be secondary in that the data were collected for other purposes yet they can be useful for tracking injuries, illnesses and deaths that occur in a defined population.

Occupational health surveillance is the tracking of workplace injuries, illnesses, hazards, and exposures. In the U. S., because there are no periodic national surveys of worker health, occupational health surveillance remains fragmented with substantial data gaps. However, the available surveillance data are used to guide efforts to improve worker safety and health and to monitor trends and progress over time [NIOSH 2013b]. Data and information derived from surveillance can be used to:

(1) guide immediate action for important cases;
(2) measure the burden of an injury, disease, or other health-related event or exposure, including changes in related factors;
(3) identify populations at risk, including new or emerging health concerns;
(4) guide the planning, implementation, and evaluation of programs to prevent and control injuries, disease, or adverse exposures;
(5) evaluate policies and practices;
(6) detect changes in health practices and the effects of the changes;
(7) prioritize the allocation of health resources;

---

[18]For a thorough explanation of public health research and non-research as defined by CDC, please see http://www.cdc.gov/od/science/integrity/docs/cdc-policy-distinguishing-public-health-research-nonresearch.pdf .

(8) describe the clinical course of disease; and
(9) provide a basis for epidemiologic research.

Workers' compensation records, most commonly administrative claims data, are used for occupational surveillance. In some states, for example California (California Labor Code) and Washington (Department of Labor and Industries), workers' compensation claims information is used to identify more hazardous industries or leading events for claims across all industries. Claims information has been used to establish priorities for loss prevention and other intervention actions [Silverstein et al. 2002; Bonauto et al. 2006; Anderson et al. 2013]. Yet other investigators have determined that workers' compensation claims data are currently inadequate to characterize occupational injuries and illnesses in particular [Rosenman et al. 2000; Azaroff et al. 2002; Utterback et al. 2012].

Formerly, workers' compensation claims information from a large number of states was collected by BLS for the Supplementary Data System (SDS), a non-representative sample of occupational injuries and illnesses. SDS contained discrepancies due to the quality of data retrieved from states and the variability of state laws on which injuries and illnesses were reported [National Research Council 1987]. The system was discontinued in the late 1980's when the Survey of Occupational Injuries and Illnesses (SOII) along with the Census of Fatal Occupational Injuries (CFOI) were being developed.

Estimating Rates
Rates of occupational injuries and illnesses require estimates of at-risk populations (a "denominator"). The denominator commonly used in the workers' compensation industry is dollars of payroll. In public health, preferred denominators for rates are numbers of people or, in the case of occupational studies, full-time equivalent (FTE) workers. Data sets used to estimate the numbers of workers within industries and/or occupations may be obtained from population household surveys such as the Current Population Survey (CPS) or the American Community Survey (ACS), or from employer establishment survey programs such as Occupational Employment Statistics (OES), Current Employment Statistics (CES), or County Business Patterns (CBP). All of these data sources have broad coverage but exclude some types of workers. The Quarterly Census of Employment and Wages (QCEW), which is nearly comprehensive and collected by states for unemployment insurance purposes does report the number of workers by establishments although it does not distinguish between full-time and part-time workers. The QCEW data may be adjusted to estimate FTEs with hours per industry data from the surveys listed above. In any case, the scope, exclusions, and restrictions on survey and state level data should be carefully examined and understood.

> Estimations of the populations at risk that are needed for rate calculations are likely to require information from record sets other than workers' compensation.

15. Public Health Regulations

Many Federal, state and local government regulations have been developed to address public health concerns. It is beyond the scope of this document to describe the myriad public health concerns that are regulated. Instead, we limit this description to those authorities where workers' compensation data may be useful. The Occupational Safety and Health Administration (OSHA) and the Mine Safety and Health Administration (MSHA) are two Federal agencies with regulatory mandates to protect the health and safety of workers in the U.S. OSHA and MSHA regulations are available through their respective Web sites and elsewhere.[19, 20] Additionally, the US Environmental Protection Agency regulates pesticide hazards for agricultural workers.[21] State and local health departments are

---

[19] http://www.osha.gov/law-regs.html
[20] http://www.msha.gov/30CFR/CFRINTRO.HTM
[21] http://www.epa.gov/agriculture/twor.html

charged with protecting the health of all residents in their jurisdictions, and some health departments are active in workplace health and safety and tracking occupational illnesses and injuries. In fiscal year 2013, NIOSH provided funds to help support occupational health and safety surveillance programs in twenty-three states.[22]

> Regulations are perceived by many as essential to the protection of public health. Individuals may not have the knowledge or resources that are required to make decisions about personal exposure to potentially hazardous materials including chemical, ergonomic, physical and biological agents.

Regulations are perceived by many as essential to the protection of public health. Individuals may not have the knowledge or resources that are required to make decisions about personal exposure to potentially hazardous materials including chemical, ergonomic, physical and biological agents. In the occupational arena, regulations are established by OSHA and MSHA to limit potential hazards through the use of interventions such as exposure limits, machine guarding, fall protection, trenching standards, medical screening and many more.

Regulations pertaining to workers' compensation are established by the individual jurisdictions including the states, territories, and the District of Columbia, and the Federal government for its own employees. The states frequently require all employers including those self-insured for workers' compensation to provide health and safety programs for their establishments. These requirements vary substantially across the jurisdictions and many are augmented by occupational safety and health requirements in departments of labor or similar agencies. Carrier-based loss prevention programs often assist employers in the recognition and control of hazards for which regulations apply. In addition to the insurance claims and medical information, records for these mandated activities may be useful for occupational safety and health research and surveillance.

> In some states, for example California and Washington, the workers' compensation claims information is used to identify more hazardous industries or leading events for claims across all industries.

16. Breaking through Barriers

Despite its limitations, research organizations, state-based surveillance programs, and workers' compensation agencies and associations have used claims data for research and surveillance purposes. Collaborations have been mostly within states due to problems with combining data from multiple jurisdictions. Additional collaborations would create further opportunities to use workers' compensation records and related information to prevent occupational injuries, illnesses and fatalities.

Overcoming some of the limitations would be possible with more systematic collection and analysis of workers' compensation data across industries and occupations. Further standardization of data elements and coding schemes such as universal adoption of ICD medical codes and ICD-E external cause of injury codes would be beneficial. Development of additional computer-based record systems would provide greater opportunities for more informative data collection and interpretation. Advances in auto-coding of data by computer systems, which rely on standard codes, would reduce the number of errors and missing

---

[22] The NIOSH funded surveillance programs in 2013 exist in the following states: California, Colorado, Connecticut, Florida, Georgia, Illinois, Iowa, Kentucky, Louisiana, Maryland, Massachusetts, Michigan, Minnesota, Nebraska, New Hampshire, New Jersey, New Mexico, New York, North Carolina, Oregon, Texas, Washington, and Wisconsin.

data from the workers' compensation insurance records. Effective searching of unstructured text fields has also improved [Lehto et al. 2009; Patel et al. 2012; Bertke et al. 2013].

Although systematic data analysis within a carrier's operations contributes to risk management goals and client service, the information is not readily available to public health organizations. When made available, practitioners and researchers have used claims data for epidemiologic studies, to identify hazards, assess the effectiveness of controls, assign priorities for limited resources, and evaluate intervention programs.

Additional information on evaluations of workplace safety and health programs, hazard monitoring and hazard exposure data, and observations of worksites are types of loss prevention information that could be standardized and made more useful for research and surveillance purposes. Over the past century and more, carrier-based and state agency workers' compensation programs have used data to identify and evaluate risks for specific hazards across industry sectors.

When systematically available, workers' compensation data has been used extensively for occupational safety and health research and surveillance [NIOSH 2010; Utterback et al. 2012; NIOSH 2013a] and they have supplemented the surveillance information available from other occupational resources.[23] This primer provides background information for those interested in utilizing workers' compensation data for prevention purposes.

---

[23]Descriptions of many data sources used for occupational surveillance may be accessed at http://wwwn.cdc.gov/niosh-survapps/Gateway/DataSources.aspx.

References

American Association of State Compensation Insurance Funds [2007]. State Funds: Their Role in Workers' Compensation, [http://www.aascif.org/public/1.1.1_history.htm] Accessed on November 8, 2013.

Anderson NJ, Bonauto DK, Adams D [2013]. Prioritizing Industries for Occupational Injury and Illness Prevention and Research, Washington State Workers' Compensation Claims Data, 2002-2010. Washington State Department of Labor and Industries Technical Report Number 64-1-2013 [http://www.lni.wa.gov/Safety/Research/Files/bd_3F.pdf]. Accessed on November 8, 2013.

Azaroff LS, Levenstein C, Wegman DH [2002]. Occupational injury and illness surveillance: Conceptual filters explain underreporting. Am J Pub Health 92:1421-1429.

Bertke SJ, Meyers AR, Wurzelbacher SJ, Bell J, Lampl ML, Robins D [2012]. Development and evaluation of a Naïve Bayesian model for coding causation of workers' compensation claims. J Safety Res 43(5-6):327-32.

Biddle J, Roberts K, Rosenman KD, Welch EM [1998]. What percentage of workers with work-related illnesses receive workers' compensation benefits? J Occup Environ Med 40:325-331.

Boden LI, Biddle EA, Spieler EA [2001]. Social and economic impacts of workplace illness and injury: Current and future directions for research. Am J Ind Med 40:398-402.

Boden L, Ozonoff A [2008]. Capture-recapture estimates of nonfatal workplace injuries and illnesses. Annals Epidem 18:500-506.

Bonauto DK, Silverstein BA, Adams D, Foley M [2006]. Prioritizing industries for occupational injury and illness prevention and research. J Occup Environ Med 48:840-851.

Burton JF [2004]. A primer on workers' compensation, Workers' Compensation Policy Review. Nov/Dec 2004 [http://workerscompresources.com/wp-content/uploads/2012/11/ND04A.pdf]. Accessed November 7, 2013.

California Labor Code, Sections 6314.1, 6354 and 6355 [http://www.dir.ca.gov/doshpol/P&PC-19.html]. Accessed on November 7, 2013

CDC [2010]. Distinguishing public health research and public health nonresearch, CDC-SA-2010-02, July 29, 2010 [http://www.cdc.gov/od/science/integrity/docs/cdc-policy-distinguishing-public-health-research-nonresearch.pdf]. Accessed November 7, 2013.

Cocchiarella L, Anderson GBJ, eds. [2001] Guides to the Evaluation of Permanent Impairment. 5th ed. Chicago, Ill: American Medical Association.

Courtney TK [2010]. Workers' compensation data utilization in injury prevention research at the Liberty Mutual Research Institute for Safety. In: Proceedings of Use of Workers' Compensation Data for Occupational Injury and Illness Prevention. Utterback DF, Schnorr TM eds. Cincinnati, OH. National Institute for Occupational Safety and Health; DHHS (NIOSH) Pub No. 2010-152. pp. 49-53.

Dembe AE [1995]. Alternative approaches for incorporating safety into state workers' compensation reform legislation. J Insurance Regulation 13:445-450.

Department of Health and Human Services, Health Information Privacy, [2003] Disclosures for Workers' Compensation Purposes 45 C.F.R. Sect. 164.512(l) [http://www.hhs.gov/ocr/privacy/hipaa/understanding/coveredentities/workerscomp.html]. Accessed on November 12, 2013.

Department of Health and Human Services [2013]. Workers' compensation settlements and payments [http://www.medicare.gov/supplement-other-insurance/how-medicare-works-with-other-insurance/who-pays-first/workers-comp-payments.html]. Accessed on November 12, 2013

Environmental Protection Agency [2013]. Worker Protection Standard for Agricultural Pesticides. [http://www.epa.gov/agriculture/twor.html]. Accessed on November 12, 2013.

Fan ZJ, Bonauto DK, Foley MP, Silverstein BA [2006]. Underreporting of work-related injury or illness to workers' compensation: individual and industry factors. J Occup Environ Med 48:914-922.

Fishback PV [2013]. Workers' Compensation. EH.net, [http://eh.net/encyclopedia/workers-compensation/]. Accessed on November 12, 2013

Florida Division of Workers' Compensation [2012]. 2011 Division of Workers' Compensation Annual Report. [http://www.myfloridacfo.com/wc/pdf/DWC-Annual-Report-2011.pdf]. Accessed May 10, 2013

Guyton GP [1999]. A Brief History of Workers' Compensation. Iowa Orthop J. 19: 106–110. [http://www.ncbi.nlm.nih.gov/pmc/articles/PMC1888620/]. Accessed on November 12, 2013.

Hakimzadeh S, Cohn D [2007]. English usage among Hispanics in the United States, Pew Research Hispanic Center; Nov 29, 2007. [http://www.pewhispanic.org/2007/11/29/iv-workplace-and-home/]. Accessed on November 7, 2013.

Hunt HA [2003-2004]. Benefit adequacy in state workers' compensation programs. Social Security Bulletin. 65(4):24-30.

International Association of Industrial Accident Boards and Commissions [2004]. A History of the IAIABC, 90th Annual Convention Edition http://www.iaiabc.org/files/Resources/2006HistoryofIAIABC.pdf. Accessed May 12, 2013

International Association of Industrial Accident Boards and Commissions [2013]. EDI Implementation Guides. [http://www.iaiabc.org/i4a/pages/index.cfm?pageid=3339]. Accessed on November 12, 2013.

Kiselica D, Sibson B, Green-McKenzie J [2004] Workers' compensation: a historical review and description of a legal and social insurance system. Clin Occup Environ Med. May;4(2):v, 237-47.

Lehto M, Marucci-Wellman H, Corns H [2009]. Bayesian methods: A useful tool for classifying injury narratives into cause groups. Inj Prev Aug;15(4):259-65.

Leigh JP [2011]. Economic burden of occupational injury and illness in the United States. Milbank Q 89:728-72.

Leigh JP, Marcin JP [2012]. Workers' compensation benefits and shifting costs for occupational injury and illness. J Occup Environ Med 54:445-450.

Lipscomb HJ, Dement JM, Silverstein BA, Cameron W, Glazner JE [2009]. Who is paying the bills? Health care costs for musculoskeletal back disorders, Washington State carpenters, 1989 – 2003. J Occup Environ Med 51:1185-1192.

Mine Health and Safety Administration [2013]. Title 30 CFR Mineral Resources Parts 1 through 199. [http://www.msha.gov/30CFR/CFRINTRO.HTM]. Accessed November 12, 2013.

Missouri Department of Labor and Industrial Relations [2012]. Report of Injury. [http://labor.mo.gov/DWC/Forms/WC-1-EDI-AI.pdf]. Accessed November 12, 2013.

Morin JF, Utterback DF, Shor G, Welsh L, Bogyo TJ, Wurzelbacher SJ [2013]. Workers' compensation loss prevention information and interventions. Submitted for publication

National Commission on State Workmen's Compensation Laws [1972]. The Report of the National Commission on State Workmen's Compensation Laws. Washington DC: Government Printing Office. [http://www.workerscompresources.com/National_Commission_Report/national_commission_report.htm]. Accessed on November 12, 2013.

National Research Council [1987]. Counting injuries and illnesses in the workplace: Proposals for a better system. Pollack ES and Keimig DG eds. National Academy Press; Washington DC.

Nave M, Veltri A [2004]. Effect of loss control services on reported injury incidents. J Safety Res 35:39-46.

NIOSH [2013a]. Proceedings of Use of Workers' Compensation Data for Occupational Safety and Health, Utterback DF, Schnorr TM eds. Cincinnati, OH; National Institute for Occupational Safety and Health; DHHS (NIOSH) Pub No. 2013-147.

NIOSH [2013b]. Topic Page: Surveillance Program. [http://www.cdc.gov/niosh/programs/surv/]. Accessed November 7, 2013.

NIOSH [2010]. Proceedings of Use of Workers' Compensation Data for Occupational Injury and Illness Prevention. Utterback DF, Schnorr TM eds. Cincinnati, OH. National Institute for Occupational Safety and Health; DHHS (NIOSH) Pub No. 2010-152.

Occupational Safety and Health Administration [2013]. OSHA Law & Regulations. [http://www.osha.gov/law-regs.html]. Accessed November 12, 2013.

Oklahoma Insurance Department [2013]. Self-Funded Health Care Plans/Self-Insured Employers. [https://www.ok.gov/oid/Consumers/Insurance_Basics/ERISA_Information.html]. Accessed November 7, 2013.

Oleinick A, Zaidman B [2004]. Methodologic issues in the use of workers' compensation database for the study of work injuries with day away from work. I. Sensitivity of case ascertainment. Am J Ind Med 45:260-274.

Oregon [2013]. 2012 Oregon Workers' Compensation Premium Rate Ranking Summary. [http://actprod.cbs.state.or.us/iportal/report_catalog.html]. Accessed on November 7, 2013

O'Leary P, Boden LI, Seabury SA, Ozonoff A, Scherer E [2012]. Workplace injuries and the take-up of Social Security disability benefits. Social Security Bulletin 72(3):1-17.

Ostbye T, Dement JM, Krause KM [2007]. Obesity and workers' compensation: Results from the Duke Health and Safety Surveillance System. Arch Intern Med 167:766-73.

Patel MD, Rose KM, Owens CR, Bang H, Kaufman JS [2012]. Performance of automated and manual coding systems for occupational data: A case study of historical records. Am J Ind Med 55(3):228-31.

Restrepo T, Shuford H [2011]. Workers' compensation and the aging workforce. National Council on Compensation Insurance, Boca Raton, FL. [https://www.ncci.com/documents/2011_Aging_Workforce_Research_Brief.pdf]. Accessed on November 7, 2013.

Rosenman KD, Gardiner JC, Wang J, Biddle J, Hogan A, Reilly MJ, Roberts K, Welch E [2000]. Why most workers with occupational repetitive trauma do not file for workers' compensation. J Occup Environ Med 42:25-34.

Ryan M [2013]. Risk management and loss control industry trends. Presented at: E&S 2013 Loss Control Executive Forum, March 5, 2013 [http://www.iso.com/Conferences/Loss-Control-Forum/Home.html?blogclick%20E&S%20Forum%20link]. Accessed on November 7, 2013.

Scherzer T, Wolfe N [2008]. Barriers to workers' compensation and medical care for injured personal assistance services workers. Home Health Care Serv Q 27:37-58.

Schmid F, Laws C, Montero M [2012]. Indemnity benefit duration and obesity. National Council on Compensation Insurance, Boca Raton, FL. [https://www.ncci.com/documents/Obesity-2012.pdf]. Accessed on November 7, 2013.

Sengupta I, Reno V, Burton JF, Baldwin M [2012]. Workers' Compensation: Benefits, Coverage, and Costs, 2010, National Academy of Social Insurance, Washington DC.

Shuford H [2013]. The role of professional employer organizations in workers compensation: Evidence of workplace safety and reporting. In: Proceedings of Use of Workers' Compensation Data for Occupational Safety and Health Workshop. Utterback DF, Schnorr TM eds. NIOSH Pub. No. 2013-147. pp. 51 – 56.

Shuford H, Restrepo T, Beaven N, Leigh JP [2009]. Trends in components of medical spending within workers' compensation: Results from 37 states combined. J Occup Environ Med 51:232-238.

Silverstein BA, Viikari-Juntura E, Kalat J [2002]. Use of a prevention index to identify injuries at high risk for work-related musculoskeletal disorders of the neck, back and upper extremity in Washington State. Am J Ind Med 41:149-169.

Smith CK, Silverstein BA, Bonauto DK, Adams D, Fan ZJ [2010]. Temporary workers in Washington State. Am J Ind Med 53: 135-145.

Spieler E [1994]. Perpetuating risk? Workers' compensation and the persistence of occupational injuries, 31 Houston Law Rev. 119-264. Excerpts reprinted in Employment Law (Rothstein M, Leibman L, eds.); 1995 Workers' Compensation Yearbook (Burton, JF Jr. ed. 1994).

Spieler EA, Burton JF [2012]. The lack of correspondence between work-related disability and receipt of workers' compensation benefits. Am J Ind Med 55:487-505.

Spielholz P, Cullen J, Smith C, Howard N, Silverstein BA, Bonauto DK [2008]. Assessment of perceived injury risks and priorities among truck drivers and trucking companies in Washington State. J Safety Res 39:569-576.

Thacker SB, Qualters JR, Lee LM [2012]. Public health surveillance in the United States: Evolution and challenges. MMWR (Suppl) 61(03):3-9.

Thamann D, Reitz D [2000]. Workers' Compensation Guide, Interpretation and Analysis, The National Underwriter Company, Cincinnati, OH.

Trogdon JG, Finkelstein EA, Hylands T, Dellea PS, Kamal-Bahl SJ [2008]. Indirect costs of obesity: A review of the current literature. Obes Rev 9(5):489-500.

U.S. Bureau of Labor Statistics [2012]. News Release: Nonfatal occupational injuries and illnesses requiring days away from work, 2011. Washington DC. November 8, 2012. [http://www.bls.gov/news.release/osh2.nr0.htm]. Accessed on June 11, 2013

U.S. Chambers of Commerce [2012]. 2011 Analysis of Workers' Compensation Laws. Washington DC. (Updated annually in July of subsequent year)

Utterback DF, Schnorr TM, Silverstein BA, Spieler EA, Leamon TB, Amick BC [2012]. Occupational health and safety surveillance and research using workers' compensation data. J Occup Environ Med 54:171-176.

Washington State Department of Labor and Industries [2012]. Division of Occupational Safety and Health, Directive 2.10: Programmed inspection and visit activities, January 5, 2012. [http://www.lni.wa.gov/Safety/Rules/Policies/PDFs/WRD210.pdf]. Accessed on November 7, 2013.

Willborn SL, Schwab SJ, Burton JF, Lester GLL [2012]. Employment Law: Cases and Materials. LexisNexis, New Providence, NJ.. p. 881.

Winslow, Charles-Edward Amory [1920]. The untilled fields of public health. Science 51(1306): 23–33.

Wurzelbacher SJ, Meyers AR, Bertke SJ, Lampl M, Robins DR, Bushnell PT, Tarawneh A, Childress D, Turnes J [2013]. Comparison of cost valuation methods for workers compensation. In: Proceedings of Use of Workers' Compensation Data for Occupational Safety and Health Workshop. Utterback DF, Schnorr TM eds. NIOSH Pub. No. 2013-147. pp.147-151.

Appendix A: Workers' Compensation Primer Glossary and Other Industry Terms

actuary – one who calculates insurance premiums, reserves and dividends

adjuster – see claims adjuster

appeal – right of an individual who received an adverse decision to seek review by a higher authority

assigned risk – an insured entity that would normally be rejected by commercial insurance carriers in the voluntary market but is designated for coverage by state law

audit – examination and verification of employer records on payroll

basic premium – portion of a standard retrospective insurance premium that covers administrative costs, fees and commissions

broker – business that sells insurance coverage to employers; may represent a number of insurance carriers

captive – insurance provider for a single business organization that is owned by that organization

carrier – organization acting as an insurer

carve-outs – labor/management agreements for insurance coverage of occupational injuries and illnesses (has various other meanings in the insurance industry as a whole)

case manager – insurer representative that oversees medical treatments for injury or illness claims

claim – application for insurance benefits due to occupational injury or illness

claim disallowance – insurer rejection of a claim for medical treatment or indemnity costs

claimant – person making a demand for payment of benefits

claims adjuster – insurer representative who investigates claims for authenticity and settlements

claims initiator – person who completes the initial claim form for compensation

deductible – a type of workers' compensation insurance policy for which the initial loss to some specified limit is not reimbursed by insurance payment, i.e. the risk is retained by employer

disability – condition that curtails a person's ability to carry on normal pursuits

dividend plan – a type of workers' compensation insurance policy for which the insured may receive funds back (a dividend) if losses are less than anticipated

doctor's first report – initial claimant evaluation by physician which is required in some states

Electronic Data Interchange – developed several standard claim data reporting forms and was fostered by the IAIABC

exclusive funds – state-sponsored workers' compensation insurance in jurisdictions where private insurance is not allowed

exclusive remedy – in workers' compensation, the only recourse for worker injuries and illnesses

experience modification factor – multiplier adjustment to employer's premium based on prior claims history in comparison with the average experience of the risk class, may be greater than or less than unity

first report of injury – initial form completed by claims initiator with detailed information on the claimant, employer, nature of injury, event description, and anticipated medical treatment needs

groups – similar industry employers that combine to share risks and insurance coverage; also may be employees that are covered under single insurance policy, e.g. group health insurance

guaranteed cost – a type of workers' compensation insurance policy where the premium is the only cost to the employer

impairment – alteration of an individual's health status; a deviation from normal in a body part or organ system and its functioning (Cocchiarella and Anderson 2001)

incurred losses – paid plus reserved claim costs, including medical and indemnity; experience modification ratings are based on incurred costs

indemnity payments – compensation for lost work time claim paid to covered injured or ill workers to partially replace lost wages

independent medical examiner – registered medical practitioners who provide impartial medical assessments

loss control – see loss prevention

loss development factor – prediction of future payments on open claims

loss prevention – actions to limit risk through hazard recognition and abatement and safety and health program evaluation; also known as loss control

loss ratio – insured losses divided by premiums earned in a given period

loss reduction – activities to limit financial losses and disability after a claim is filed for an injury or illness; also known as medical or disability management

loss runs – employer-based information on prior claims experience

lost work days – accrual of time away from work due to an occupational injury or illness

managed care – enrolled medical services that focuses on care utilization and costs

manual rate – published rates, established by rating bureaus, for insured groups based on average costs for the group

medical only claim – workers' compensation claim for medical treatment expenses and does not include lost work days meeting the minimum lost time requirement for indemnity payments

medical review board – state sanctioned group of medical practitioners that provides independent medical expertise on appropriate treatments, disability determination, and other science-based criteria

Medicare set-aside – allocation in a claim settlement to pay future medical expenses that would have been paid by Medicare

monopolistic funds – see exclusive funds

mutual insurance company – organization that issues insurance policies and is owned by its policyholders

net premium – total insurance premium after adjustments for experience modification and discounts

pools – multiple meanings but usually a collection of groups that share insurance coverage

professional employer organization (PEO) – firm that hires a client company's employees, becoming the policy holder of record for workers' compensation; this arrangement results in co-employment

pure premium – portion of manual rate that covers anticipated losses and loss adjustment expenses

rating bureau – state sanctioned private group that establishes permitted manual rates for insurance premiums

reciprocal group – association of employer entities that mutually share risks of economic losses

re-insurance – insurance purchased by an insurance carrier to limit risks

reserve funds – accounting liability for the current value of future expected costs on a claim

residual market – portion of employers unable to obtain insurance coverage in the voluntary market

retrospective rating – a type of workers' compensation insurance policy where the premium is based on the actual insured losses during the policy term

return-to-work – program to assist injured workers regain employment after a claim has been filed

risk group – see groups

risk retention – portion of possible future liability that is not covered by an insurance policy

scheduled benefit – pre-determined amount of payment for specified loss such as an amputation

Second Injury Fund – insurance provided for previously disabled workers

self-insured – a type of workers' compensation insurance policy where the employer is responsible for its own losses associated with required risk coverage

single payer – for health insurance, a single entity, generally a government agency, is responsible for all insured costs

state funds – state government offered mandatory insurance; may be exclusive (monopolistic) in a few states or competitive in yet other states

subrogation – recovery of claim expenses from another responsible party

Supplemental Data System – survey of workers' compensation claims information by Bureau of Labor Statistics in the 1970's and 1980's prior to the Survey of Occupational Injuries and Illnesses and the Census of Fatal Occupational Injuries

surety bond – financially backed guarantee to reimburse third party losses

surveillance – ongoing systematic collection, analysis, and interpretation of health data essential to the planning, implementation, and evaluation of public health practices, closely integrated with the timely dissemination of these data to those who need to know

third-party administrator – insurance businesses that provide services to employers, brokers, insurers, and groups related to workers' compensation claims

underwriter – one who selects risks to be solicited or rates the acceptability of risks

underwriting – to be responsible for financial losses in accordance with an insurance policy

uninsured employer fund – state funds to cover losses when employer has failed to obtain required insurance

Unit Statistical Report – information on workers' compensation loss experiences reported to a rating agency

value – estimates of current or future liability costs on a claim

voluntary market – competitive market for workers' compensation insurance that exists in all but the 4 exclusive fund states

Appendix B: Preparing for Engagement

In preparation for contacting the workers' compensation data custodian, one should consider several issues and evaluate some available resources. For example, one should visit the Web site for the workers' compensation program in the state to evaluate the available information such as annual reports and reporting forms. In addition, the Web sites have links to applicable statutes and regulations with explanatory guides for injured workers and their employers. Researchers and public health practitioners may also want to think about the issues below prior to approaching potential collaborating organizations who are workers' compensation data custodians. If the state workers' compensation Web sites does not provide specific information on their requirements, these issues may be addressed in direct communications with a knowledgeable agency official.

Study Background Questions

What are the proposed project concept and time commitments? Might provide examples from other jurisdictions
- Surveillance – ongoing analysis of longitudinal data
- Etiologic research – may be time limited relationship but usually longitudinal data

What data sources may be needed for the project?
- Public agencies – do they have a research unit or other organization with shared interest/mission?
- Private – if restricted, can they share de-identified data, are they comprehensive?

Are there specific legal restrictions on data availability from state agencies?

Can data be examined or explored prior to collaboration commitment?

What are the possible mutual benefits for the collaborating organizations?
- Examine their existing products
- Review examples from other jurisdictions (e.g. Florida Annual Report)
- Reinforce experience with confidential handling of personal and other sensitive information
- Think about realistic needs for future information, assistance and review

How are data stored and what formats are used?
- Electronic: on line or downloaded (CD, DVD, hard drives, encryption?)
- Hard copy
- Incomplete data and historical gaps in data
- Denominator (population) data available for rate estimation (unemployment insurance agencies)?

Which, if any, standardized data coding systems and which versions are used (e.g. WCIO, OIICS, NCCI, NAICS, ICD E-codes)?

Is a data dictionary available?

Are narrative fields part of the records that may require data mining?

What are the proposed agreements for clearance of articles, reports and other products?

Other State Coverage Questions

If the state publishes an annual report, what kind of information is captured in the report?

What exclusion criteria are used to decide which employers need to provide workers' compensation coverage for workers? For example
- Minimum employer size*
- Industry sector (e.g. agriculture)*
- Familial relationship of the employee with the employer*
- Self-employed workers*
- Corporate officers*

Are separate rules written for industries such as agriculture, construction or mining?

Does the state offer workers' compensation insurance plans? If yes, for which employers?

Which employers, if any, are allowed to self-insure in the state?*

Does NCCI or another rating bureau collect standardized data from insurance carriers in the state?

Does the state require private insurance companies to write coverage for residual market employers?

Are employers in the state allowed to form groups or pools to obtain insurance in the voluntary markets?

Are employers in the state allowed to combine to create a self-insured entity?

Are carve-out arrangements permitted in the state?

What automatic, Web-based or telemetric reporting systems are used in the state?

Who can file a first report of injury?

What requirements exist related to managed care organizations in the state?*

What requirements govern the choice of treating physicians in the state?*

What requirements exist related to vocational rehabilitation in the state?*

What requirements restrict treatment options in the state?*

Has the state imposed any time or cost limits on compensation for disabled workers? If yes, what are they?*

*Answers to these questions can be found in the annual "Analysis of Workers' Compensation Laws" produced by U.S. Chambers of Commerce

www.ingramcontent.com/pod-product-compliance
Lightning Source LLC
Chambersburg PA
CBHW081752170526
45167CB00009B/4009